Endorsements for

"All I can say about *Getting into Your Pants* is well-done! [With its] conversational writing style, it's a fun and easy read. Bett[er yet, it's a] common sense program with three simple rules. Just follo[w the rules], and you will lose weight while improving your health."
—Alan Goldhamer, D.C., co-author of *The Pleasure Trap*

"Follow Dr. Leslie's 10+10 for Life® and all those frustrations from those restrictive diets that never worked will disappear, right along with that weight. Refreshingly, Dr. Leslie masterfully cuts through the confusion and offers a simple solution for losing weight – the right way. And big bonus: she's right on with her food facts. Instead of listening to the food industries' slick marketing ads masquerading as nutrition information, take it from an intelligent, experienced woman who knows her stuff. But even better, she walks her talk. Dr. Leslie is a shining example of glowing health and vibrancy."
—George Eisman, Registered Dietician, author of *The Most Noble Diet* and *Don't Let Your Diet Add to Your Cancer Risk*

"Dr. Van Romer shares her powerful formula for permanent weight loss and optimal health. *Getting into Your Pants* is a book that will motivate and inspire people to make positive changes in their health and their life."
—Joel Fuhrman, M.D., author of *Eat to Live* and *Eat for Health*

"Dr. Van Romer's book, *Getting into Your Pants*, extends the amazing broad-based effects of a plant-based diet to that all-important need - losing weight and keeping it off. I highly recommend it."
—T. Colin Campbell, Ph.D., author of *The China Study* and Jacob Gould Schurman Professor Emeritus of Nutritional Biochemistry at Cornell University

"*Getting into Your Pants* is an entertaining read and a great review of the ten thousand reasons you need to follow a low-fat vegan diet."
—John McDougall, M.D., author of *The McDougall Program – Twelve Days to Dynamic Health* and *The McDougall Program for a Healthy Heart*

"This is NOT a book! This is an opportunity… an opportunity to live longer, live healthier and live in the body you've always dreamed of. Dr. Leslie's brilliant strategies will liberate you from the life-threatening disease of dieting. In each powerful lesson you'll effortlessly lose the fat and keep it off forever. This opportunity will save your life!"
—Dr. Tony Palermo, Success Coach

Getting *into* Your Pants

Copyright © 2008 by Leslie Van Romer

All rights reserved. No part of this book may be used or reproduced in any manner whatsoever without prior written consent of the author, except as provided by the United States of America copyright law.

Published by Advantage, Charleston, South Carolina.
Member of Advantage Media Group.

ADVANTAGE is a registered trademark and the Advantage colophon is a trademark of Advantage Media Group, Inc.

Printed in the United States of America.

ISBN: 978-1-59932-073-1
LCCN: 2008921745

> Most Advantage Media Group titles are available at special quantity discounts for bulk purchases for sales promotions, premiums, fundraising, and educational use. Special versions or book excerpts can also be created to fit specific needs.
>
> For more information, please write: Special Markets, Advantage Media Group, P.O. Box 272, Charleston, SC 29402 or call 1.866.775.1696.

Getting *into* Your Pants

Add 10 + 10 to Lose Weight — for LIFE!

PlayBook | Your Companion Guide to *Getting into Your Pants*... lickety-split

Dr. Leslie Van Romer

Illustrations by Scott Diggs Underwood

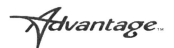

Warning: Disclaimer

The information in this book is not intended to diagnose or treat any condition or disease or to substitute for competent medical advice for your specific problems. If you are taking medications or experiencing any health problems, including, but not limited to, type 1 and type 2 diabetes, consult your health care practitioner before making dietary changes. If transitioning to weight-loss, health-supporting, and disease-fighting eating habits is safe for you, ask your practitioner to partner with you by monitoring your progress with routine check-ups and blood work.

Contents

Introduction	"But, Mooooom, I Hate Those Pants"	9
Chapter 1	Turning "Those Pants" into "Your Pants"	15
Chapter 2	Stuck in Big-Girl Pants	33
Chapter 3	Yo-Yoing In and Out of Your Pants	19
Chapter 4	"Mirror, Mirror on the Wall, Make My Pants Fit after All"	23
Chapter 5	Add "10+10" to Wiggle into Your Pants	27
Chapter 6	Breakfast: Morning Delights for Skinnier Pants What's up for breakfast?	31
Chapter 7	The Nooner: Slipping OUT of Your Pants What's up for lunch?	35
Chapters 8 & 9	Dinner: Shifting to Those Pants & Let's Drink to Your Pants What's up for dinner? What's up for beverages?	39
Chapter 10	21 "Big Buts" between You and Your Pants	45
Chapter 11	Protein, Plants, and Pants "But where do I get my protein?"	49
Chapter 12	The 20-Carb Solution into Your Pants "But don't carbs make me fat?"	53

Chapter 13	Stop the Fats to Drop Your Pants (Size)	57
	"But isn't olive oil a good fat?"	
Chapter 14	Dairy's Dirty Underpants	61
	"If I don't drink milk, where do I get my calcium?"	
Chapter 15	Panting in Your Pants	65
	"Yeah, but I hate to exercise."	
Chapter 16	Seven Sneaky Sisters Stealing Your Pants	69
Chapter 17	Part I - The First Step into Your Pants	71
	"How do I get started?"	
	Part II - Building Your Dream House	80
Addendum I	7 Steps to Stay in Those Pants	87
Addendum II	10 Top 10+10 Tips	89
Addendum III	A 10+10 Food Day In-A-Glance	91
Addendum IV	The 4 Most Common Questions and the Commonsense Answers	93
	(Protein, Calcium, Carbs, and Fats)	
Addendum V	Charts	96
	Weight Chart for Women	
	Weight Chart for Men	
	Body Mass Index	
	Risk of Diseases According to BMI and Waist Size	
	Track Your Numbers	

Introduction

Hello, my friend. Welcome to your personal *PlayBook,* your companion guide to *Getting into Your Pants* – lickety split. The point is this: the harder you play, the quicker you will lose weight and build your body-dream-come-true. The sooner you can prance in those cuter-than-heck pants, the sweeter life will be in every way. If you have fun along the way, that's even better.

Your *PlayBook* is a valuable, practical tool to help you get the most from *Getting into Your Pants*. It will help you create a doable weight-loss, body-best eating plan that works for you – not just for the short sprint of a few weeks or months, but for the long haul of your life. You don't need to be perfect (because none of us are). You just need to make enough good choices to gradually shed those layers and transition to the next level – one baby step at a time. You can do that!

Your reward for your effort: the thrill of getting into your pants, as well as a whole lot of other benefits, like more energy, more enthusiasm for life, more free time, fewer aches and pains, fewer meds, freedom from food bondage, and just feeling good about yourself.

I suggest you read *Getting into Your Pants* and complete your *Pants PlayBook* one chapter at a time. Before diving into each chapter in *Getting into Your Pants*, review the questions in the companion chapter in your *PlayBook*. That way, as you read each chapter in *Pants*, you will be thinking about how to answer the reciprocal questions in your *PlayBook*. If you've already read *Getting into Your Pants*, all the better. Now go back through the book and complete your *PlayBook,* chapter by chapter.

Thinking, self-searching, honesty, and writing will be hugely helpful in creating clear intentions, doable goals, and a gentle, but distinct, food and lifestyle shift that will get you into those pants.

It goes without saying that the more time and thought you put into this process, the more satisfied you will be with yourself in the end.

So, let's go for it – wiggling in those hot pants and giggling along the way.

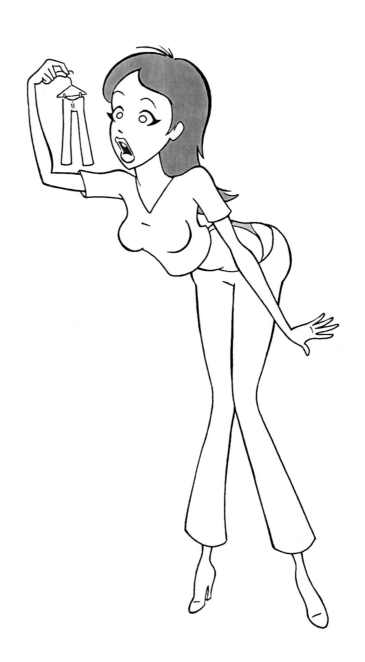

Chapter 1
Turning Those Pants into Your Pants

1. In my wildest dreams, I would like to lose _____ pounds in one year and get down to a size _____ pants, *as well as...*

   A. Eat as much food as I want
   B. Feel full and satisfied
   C. Enjoy the healthier foods that I choose to eat
   D. _____
   E. _____
   F. _____
   G. _____

2. Coming down to earth, I would *realistically* like to get down to a size _____ pants and lose _____ pounds in one year, which is only _____ pounds a month. (You will learn later what I think is a reasonable weight goal – no peeking now.)

3. *Realistically*, which of my wildest dreams in Section I can happen, along with reaching my ideal weight and pants size? (Hint: Look on pages 25-26 in *Getting into Your Pants*)

   A. _____
   B. _____
   C. _____
   D. _____
   E. _____

4. Ask yourself this all-important question: Which major food groups prevent cancer?

   The answer is _____ and _____.

   (When you get confused, think about which foods prevent cancer, heart disease, type 2 diabetes, stroke, digestive disorders, fatigue, and many more conditions and diseases. No one ever said that meat, cheese, milk, dried-up boxed cereals, and brown-colored white bread prevented cancer.)

5. Do you center your meals around fresh fruits and vegetables – your weight and disease warriors and energy and health heroes? Yes_____ No _____

6. If yes, awesome! If no, why not? Think about it for a moment and answer honestly.
   _____
   _____

WHAT YOU NOW KNOW....

You can get into your _____ while building your _____ if you:

- _____ your thinking, food _____, and lifestyle _____.
- Eat the best-for-you foods first – fresh _____ and _____.
- Believe those pants can be *your* pants by transitioning to ____ + ____ for _____ – a nutritious, simple, flexible plan tailored just for you.

Congratulations! You have already finished Chapter One. Keep up the great work. You are worth it!

"The you tomorrow is worth your effort today."

– Dr. Leslie Van Romer

Answer Key:

4. fruits, vegetables
5. yes

What You Now Know
- pants, health
- Shift, choices, habits
- fruits, vegetables
- 10,10, Life

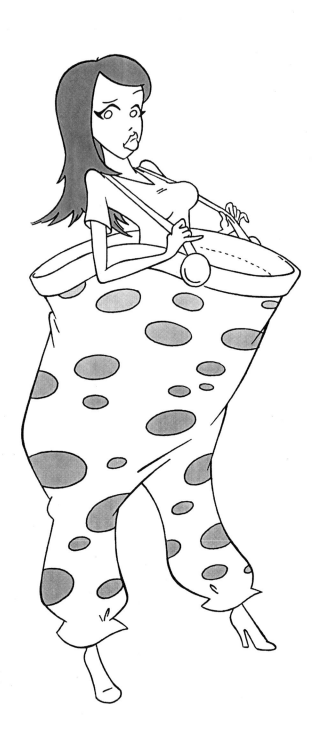

Chapter 2
Stuck in Big-Girl Pants

1. As a kid, my mother fed me the following foods, some of which were my favorites:

    Breakfast _____
    Lunch   _____
    Dinner   _____
    Snacks   _____
    Beverages _____

2. As an adult, my favorite foods are (*not* necessarily the same foods you eat):

    Breakfast _____
    Lunch   _____
    Dinner   _____
    Snacks   _____
    Beverages _____

3. About what percentage of my diet consists of my food faves listed above:
   (circle one)   100%   75%   50%   25%   10%   0%

4. I am about (circle one) 100% 75% 50% 25% 10% 0% happy with how I look and feel.

5. With all the competition from fast, easy, tasty, and "cool" foods, _____ and _____ don't stand a chance.

6. Your size _____ pants in today's sizes are actually about the same as a size _____ pants twenty years or more ago. So we're bigger than we think we are.

7. Circle the true statements:

   - 66% of Americans are overweight; 34% are obese or 30 pounds overweight.
   - Colon cancer risk increases by 3 to 4 times in obese people.
   - Eating poultry 1x a week increases the risk of colon cancer by 55%.
   - Eating poultry 4x a week increases the risk of colon cancer by 200 to 300%.
   - Smoking is still the nation's leading cause of preventable death.
   - Women with a BMI of 30 (approximately 30 pounds overweight) increase their relative risk of developing type 2 diabetes by 3000 percent – a greater correlation than the 2000 percent correlation between smoking and lung cancer.

8. I have the want and the will to do something about it – starting right now.
   Yes _____ No _____

9. Starting _____, I will reach my ideal weight and my body best by eating more _____ and _____, as well as exercising more.

WHAT YOU NOW KNOW...

- Since birth we were taught to _____ up on the _____ foods.

- Americans are clueless – we're the _____ people on the planet, killing ourselves with our own _____. We have no one to blame except _____.

- The Simple Solution for getting into your pants: eat more _____ and _____, fewer a_____ products, and less f_____, s_____, and s_____.

- Am I willing to gradually incorporate The Simple Solution into my lifestyle? Yes_____ No _____

"You didn't have a fighting chance since birth – you do now."

– Dr. Leslie Van Romer

Answer Key:

5. fruits, vegetables
6. Your pants size is really one size up than tagged compared to twenty years ago.
7. All statements are true, except overweight deaths have surpassed smoking deaths.
9. fruits, vegetables

What You Now Know
- fill, wrong
- fattest, choices, ourselves
- fruits, vegetables, animal, fat, sugar, salt

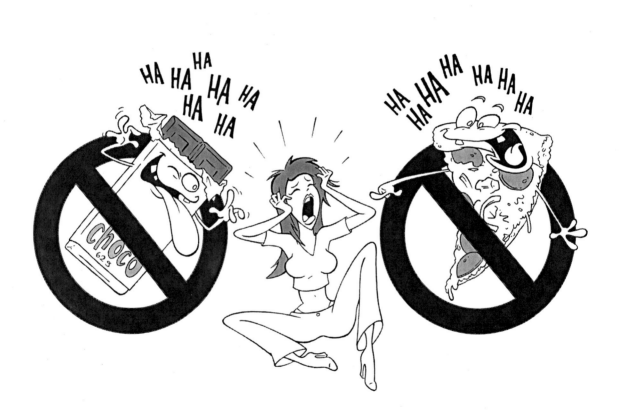

Chapter 3
Yo-Yoing In and Out of Your Pants

1. Time for a little honesty:

    A. In my lifetime, I have been on _____ diets.
    B. On my most successful diet, I lost _____ pounds in _____ months.
    C. However, I gained back _____ of those pounds.
    D. In my lifetime, I've lost approximately _____ total pounds through dieting.
    E. In my lifetime, I've gained back _____ of those pounds.
    F. When I was 20 years old, I weighed _____ pounds.
    G. I am about _____ pounds overweight right now.
    H. I would like to weigh _____ pounds right now.

2. When dieting, sooner or later I get frustrated and quit because:

    A. _____
    B. _____
    C. _____
    D. _____
    E. _____

3. Even though diets never work permanently for me, I start another diet because:

    _____

4. Diets don't work because they:

   A. don't satisfy your hunger drive, leaving you feeling _____.
   B. are too _____, making you feel trapped and deprived.
   C. emphasize too many high-fat foods and limit the important food group, _____, sourced by unrefined fresh, whole fruits and vegetables, whole grains, and legumes.
   D. increase cravings and make you feel like a _____ if you cheat or slip up.

5. 10+10 for Life® works because it:

   A. _____ you up and satisfies your hunger _____.
   B. builds flexibility into your plan, called _____ room.
   C. teaches that the only slip-up is to _____ up.
   D. _____ foods, instead of subtracting and depriving you of foods.
   E. encourages you to fill up on the _____-for-you foods first and eat the worst-for-you foods last.
   F. crushes _____, which make you nutso for certain foods.
   G. shows you how to shift your t_____, spurring you to shift your food _____ and food and lifestyle _____.

GETTING INTO YOUR PANTS

WHAT YOU NOW KNOW...

- Diets _____ work. They set you up for f_____.

- 10+10 for Life® works because you:

    - _____ up.
    - _____ your hunger drive.
    - _____ your energy.
    - _____ the best-for-you foods instead of _____, depriving, starving, and guilting.
    - crush _____ with nutrient-rich, calorie-low foods.
    - save _____ – no more counting, measuring, weighing, and fussing.
    - get into your _____ and feel _____ about yourself every step of the way.

> "You didn't fail; the diets failed you."
>
> - Dr. Leslie Van Romer

Answer Key:

4. A. hungry
    B. restrictive
    C. carbohydrates
    D. failure
5. A. fills, drive
    B. wiggle
    C. give
    D. adds
    E. best
    F. cravings
    G. thinking, choices, habits

What You Now Know
- don't, failure
- fill
- satisfy
- boost
- add, sacrificing
- cravings
- time
- pants, good

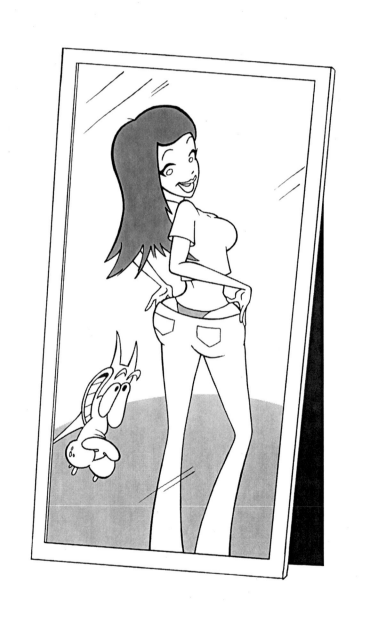

Chapter 4
Mirror, Mirror on the Wall, Make My Pants Fit after All

1. The Mirror Test

    A. When I look in the mirror, I like what I see. Yes! _____ No! _____
    B. I am sick and tired of these things about myself: Circle all that apply:

    - Looking the way I do
    - Wearing size _____ pants
    - Feeling sluggish, worn out, and old – before my time
    - Working under my potential because I don't have the energy I used to
    - Getting winded after walking a half hour or less
    - Feeling left out because I can't play with my grandkids like I want to
    - Having difficulty tying shoes because rolls get in my way
    - Taking too many pills with no end in sight
    - Fearing the same disease my mother or sister got hit with
    - Jiggling when I move – thighs, bottom, tummy, or arms
    - Avoiding intimacy with my partner because I'm embarrassed and just don't feel sexy anymore
    - Thinking/obsessing about food day in and day out
    - Feeling depressed
    - Feeling fat
    - Anything else? _____

    C. I really want it badly – to lose weight and get into those pants. Yes! ___ No ___

2. How ready am I?

   A. I'm really committed to me and ready to gradually shift my thinking, eating, exercise, and lifestyle. Yes____ No____

   B. I'm willing to learn about and then eat the best-for-me foods first each day. These are absolutely critical for me to reach my ideal weight and level of health, performance, and fitness. Yes ____ No ____

   C. I'm willing to eat the not-so-good-for-me foods last, after the best-for-me foods, automatically eating less of them without struggling. Yes____ No____

   D. I'm willing to increase my daily exercise. Yes ____ No ____

   E. I'm ready to stop making excuses for not taking control of my weight and health. Yes ____ No ____

   F. Now . . . ask yourself. Do I really want to change? Yes ____ No ____

WHAT YOU NOW KNOW...

The answers to these questions:

- How do you *really* feel about yourself – inside and out? _____

- How much do you want to weigh one year from now? _____ Five years? _____

- Do you presently eat mostly the best-for-you foods? Yes _____ No _____

- Do you exercise every day? Yes _____ No _____

- Are you really ready to commit to YOU and getting into those pants? Yes _____ No _____

"To get into your pants, you've got to really want it."

- Dr. Leslie Van Romer

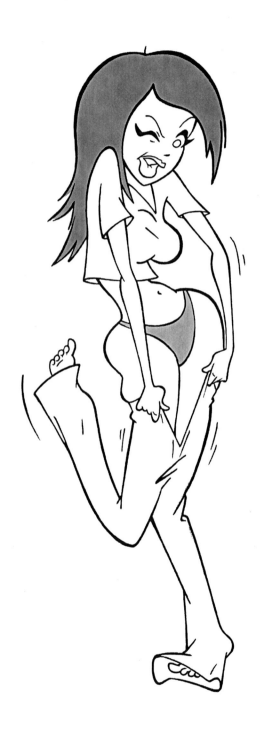

Chapter 5
Add "10+10" to Wiggle into Your Pants

1. What is 10+10 for Life®?

   A. 10+10 is a shift in thinking, food _____, lifestyle _____, **NOT** a diet.
   B. Weight warriors and health heroes are: _____ and _____.
   C. 10+10 stands for: _____ fruits and _____ vegetables a day.
   D. To lose weight, fill up on the _____-for-you foods first and then eat the _____-for-you foods last.
   E. The best-for-you foods are fresh _____ and _____.
   F. Feeling _____ is absolutely critical to losing weight.
   G. What is the big pay-off to taking the time and making the effort to change your eating and lifestyle habits? _____.

2. With every bite, ask: "Does this food feed me or deplete me?"

   A. Feed-me foods are low in salt and calories while providing all the necessary nutrients, like carbohydrates, _____, and fats, vitamins, minerals, enzymes, micronutrients, and _____, the colon sweeper.

   B. List some feed-me foods: _____
   _____
   _____
   _____

   C. Circle the feed-me foods above that you eat.

   D. Deplete-me foods typically increase weight, blood pressure, blood glucose, cholesterol, and/or triglycerides, and increase risk of disease, such as: _____, _____, _____, and _____.

E. List your favorite deplete-me foods that you may or may not eat:

_____

_____

_____

_____

F. Circle above your favorite deplete-me foods that you still eat.

3. Three 10+10 Rules

   A. _____ 10+10 to your day - _____ fruits and _____ vegetables - _____ up on 10+10 foods first.

   B. _____ eating when your brain says you are _____.

   C. _____, if you must! (80/20 Rule)

   D. Wiggle room or the 80/20 Rule means eat the best-for-you foods _____% of the time and wiggle _____% of the time. Beware! Don't _____ too much or you won't lose that jiggle.

4. The more _____ and _____ you eat every day, the more consistent you will be at steady, permanent weight loss.

WHAT YOU NOW KNOW...

- 10+10 for Life® means eating _____ whole, fresh fruits and _____ different, fresh vegetables every day.

- Which foods _____ you and which foods _____ you.

- 10+10's three simple rules to get into your pants:
  1. _____ and fill up on 10 fruits +10 vegetables every day.
  2. _____ eating when your brain tells you to.
  3. _____, if you must. Watch it! No more than 20% of the time.

- The reasonable weight loss goal of 30 pounds in a year (_____ pounds a month) will get me into the reasonable size _____ pants. Just _____ a month? I can do that!

"Wiggle a little to lose that jiggle."

- Dr. Leslie Van Romer

Answer Key:

1. A. choices, habits
   B. fruits, vegetables
   C. 10, 10
   D. best, worst
   E. fruits, vegetables
   F. full
   G. Getting into your pants
2. A. protein, fiber
   B. fresh fruits, raw vegetables, sprouts, raw, unsalted nuts, homemade juices, cooked fresh vegetables, frozen fruits, heated frozen vegetables, whole grains, beans
   D. heart disease, cancer, stroke, diabetes
   E. meat, fish, dairy products, eggs, white flour, white sugar, deserts, pastries, oils, salty snacks, fast foods, processed foods, refined foods, pizza, almost all beverages
3. A. Add, 10, 10, fill
   B. Stop, full
   C. Wiggle
   D. 80%, 20%, wiggle
4. fruits, vegetables

What You Now Know
- 10, 10
- feed, deplete
  1. Add
  2. Stop
  3. Wiggle
- 2.5, 2.5

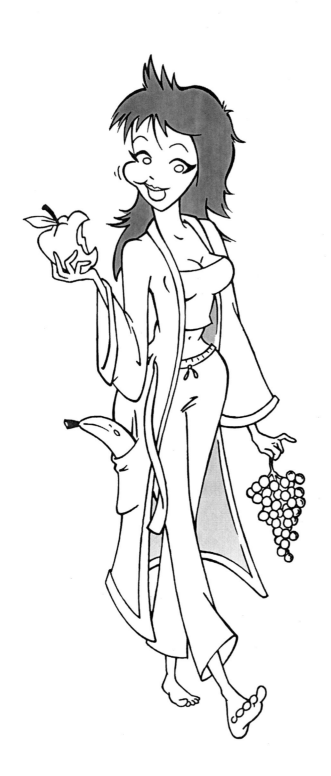

Chapter 6
Breakfast: Morning Delights for Skinnier Pants

1. Which of your morning favorites do you eat regularly? _____
   _____
   _____
   _____

2. Which of your regular morning faves are feed-me foods? _____
   _____
   _____

3. Which of your regular morning faves are deplete-me foods? _____
   _____
   _____

4. The best feed-me breakfast choices are fresh _____.

5. Eat enough fresh _____ before noon to _____ you up. Eat as many as _____ whole, fresh _____ in the morning. That many? Yes, if that's what fills you up, that many.

6. _____ eating when you get full. Throughout the morning, eat more _____ when you get hungry.

7. List the fresh fruits that you prefer and will happily graze on until noonish. (depending on the season): _____
   _____
   _____
   _____

PLAYBOOK

8. Cooked whole _____ is a good second choice feed-me breakfast food.

9. Which breakfast "big buts" are stopping you from eating feed-me breakfast foods? Example: But I'm not hungry in the morning
   A. _____
   B. _____
   C. _____

10. Are you ready to let go of your "big buts" to fill up on feed-me fresh fruits for breakfast at least 80% of the time?   Yes _____ No _____

11. List the three rules in 10+10 for Life® and give a brief explanation how to apply those three rules to breakfast.
    1. A _____:_____
    2. S _____:_____
    3. W _____:_____

WHAT YOU NOW KNOW...

- Which deplete-me foods you used to choose for breakfast.

- The ideal morning delights: up to 10 whole, fresh_____ until noon.

- Your biggest breakfast "but" that keeps you out of your pants is: _____
_____

- Are you willing to let that breakfast "big but" go and eat feed-me foods for breakfast to lose weight and build your body-best? Yes_____ No _____

Yes! One-third of your food day down, only two-thirds left to go. Go, girl, go! You can do this!

> "Fruits are the fastest fast foods —
> wash, open mouth, insert, and chew."
>
> - Dr. Leslie Van Romer

Answer Key:

4. fruits
5. fruits, fill, 10, fruits
6. Stop, fruit
7. oats
11. 1. Add: Add and fill up on up to 10 fresh fruits
    2. Stop: Stop eating fruit when brains says you're full
    3. Wiggle: 80% of time eat fresh fruit for breakfast

What You Now Know
- fruit

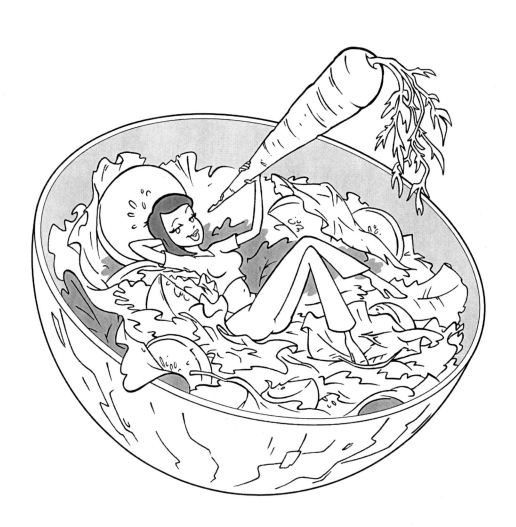

Chapter 7
The Nooner: Slipping OUT of Your Pants

1. Which lunch favorites do you eat regularly? _____
   _____
   _____

2. Which of your regular lunch faves are feed-me foods?_____
   _____

3. Which of your regular lunch faves are deplete-me foods? _____
   _____
   _____

4. The very best feed-me food for lunch is a large, ___- veggie, green-leafy _____.

5. Second best feed-me lunch choices are _____.

6. Ideally, you should add at least _____ different vegetables to your salad.

7. Create a salad and list all the ingredients that you will thoroughly enjoy. Include at least 10 different vegetables.

   A. Romaine lettuce
   B. Spinach
   C. _____
   D. _____
   E. _____
   F. _____
   G. _____
   H. _____

I. _____
J. _____
K. Black beans
L. Raw, unsalted sunflower seeds or sliced raw, unsalted almonds

8. Eat enough green-leafy, vegetable salad to ____ you up and s_____ you.

9. _____ eating when you're full. Garbage disposals are replaceable, you are not.

10. Eat feed-me foods again when you are _____.

11. Olive oil is good for only two things: more _____, which add _____ to your fat.

12. The best kind of salad dressings are _____-based with no_____, no _____ products, or chemicals.

13. Which noontime "big buts" are stopping you from eating feed-me lunch foods?

    Example: But salads don't fill me up.
    A. _____
    B. _____
    C. _____

14. Are you ready to let go of your lunch "big buts" to fill up on feed-me lunch foods at least 80% of the time?   Yes _____ No _____

15. List the three rules in 10+10 for Life® and give a brief explanation how to apply those rules to lunch.
    A. A _____:_____
    B. S _____:_____
    C. W _____:_____

WHAT YOU NOW KNOW...

- Your beloved lunch _____ usually deplete you.

- For lunch, think raw, green, color, and quantity: a large, 10-_____ salad with oil-free, dairy-free salad dressing.

- What is your biggest lunch "but" that keeps you out of your pants? _____
  _____

- Are you willing to let go of your lunch "big but" and eat feed-me foods for lunch to lose weight and build your body-best? Yes _____ No _____

"Eating vegetables is like eating air — very few calories."
- Dr. Leslie Van Romer

Answer Key:
4. 10, salad
5. vegetable sandwiches and meat-free, dairy-free, low salt soups
6. 10
8. fill, satisfy
9. Stop
10. hungry
11. calories, fat
12. water, oil, dairy
15. A. Add: a large, 10-veggie, green-leafy salad
    B. Stop: eating when brain says full and satisfied
    C. Wiggle: 80% of the time, eat 10-veggie salads for lunch; 20% wiggle

What You Now Know
- sandwiches
- veggie

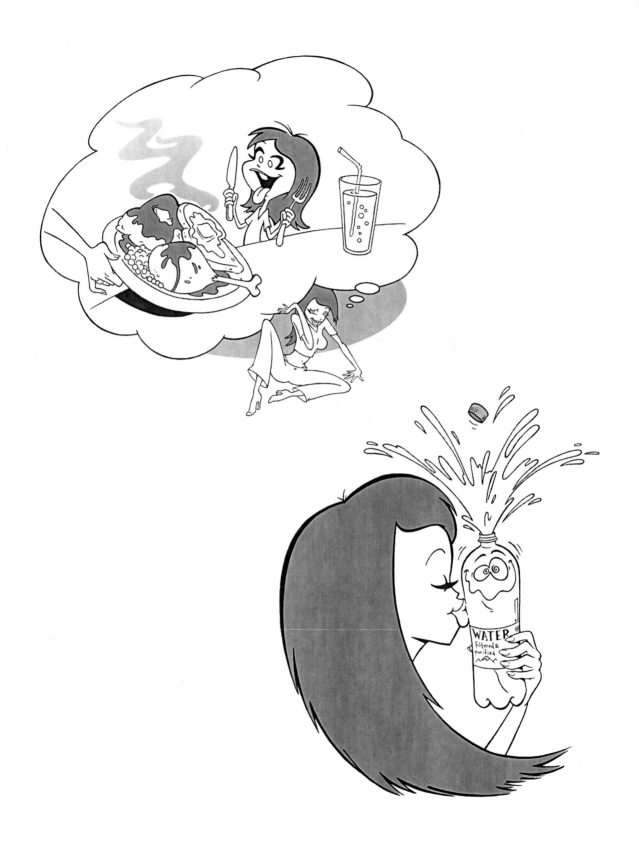

Chapters 8 & 9

Dinner: Shifting into Your Pants & Let's Drink to Your Pants

1. Which dinner favorites do you eat regularly? _____
   _____
   _____
   _____

2. Which of your regular dinner faves are feed-me foods? _____
   _____
   _____
   _____

3. Which of your regular dinner faves are deplete-me foods? _____
   _____
   _____
   _____

4. For dinner, eat in order with the very best feed-me foods first.

   - First, _____
   - Second, _____
   - Third, a more filling vegetable, like _____ or _____, whole grains, like brown _____ or legumes, like kidney or _____ beans
     Stop! Ask yourself "Am I full?" If yes, **stop** eating. If no, make a choice: more vegetables or a more traditional favorite.
   - Last, wiggle, if you must, with more traditional favorites, like _____, _____, _____, or _____.

5. Following the above 10+10 dinner line-up, create a dinner using specific foods that you will enjoy.

   First, I will eat _____.
   Second, I will eat _____.
   Third, I will eat _____.
   I will **stop** eating at this point and ask myself, "Am I _____?" If yes, I will _____ eating. If no, I will choose to eat more of the above v_____ or a traditional food favorite.

6. Which dinner "big buts" are stopping you from eating 80% feed-me dinner foods?

   Example: But my husband has to eat meat every day.
   A. _____
   B. _____
   C. _____

7. Are you ready to let go of your dinner "big buts" to fill up in order on feed-me dinner foods first, at least 80% of the time?   Yes _____ No _____

8. If yes, yippee! If no, what's stopping you?
   _____

9. List feed-me food snacks: _____

10. The two best beverage choices: _____ and homemade_____.

11. The only beverages that feed me as well as hydrate me are homemade fruit and vegetable _____.

12. All other beverages _____ you, with the exception of non-caffeinated herbal teas.

WHAT YOU NOW KNOW...

- We all love our all-American, deplete-me dinners, centered on b_____, c_____, p_____, f_____, cheese, pa_____, and brown-colored white b_____.

- To lose weight, eat dinner foods in this order:

    1. First, a 10-_____ salad with a no-oil, no-dairy, no-chemical dressing.
    2. Next, _____ of choice, like broccoli, cauliflower, green beans, asparagus.
    3. Followed by a more filling _____: potatoes, _____ potatoes, yams, winter squash (no butter, margarine, or sour cream please) *or* a whole grain, like brown rice, or legumes, like kidney beans or _____ beans.
    4. Very last, if you must: traditional American foods, like beef, chicken, pork, fish, cheese, or pasta.

- What is your biggest dinner "but" that keeps you out of your pants? _____ _____.

- Are you willing to let your dinner "big but" go to eat feed-me foods for dinner to lose weight and build your body-best?   Yes____ No ____

- Beverages contribute about _____% of daily calories consumed, translating into extra _____ that keeps you out of your pants.

- Most beverages _____ you with sugar, sugar substitutes, protein, colorings, preservatives, chemicals, alcohol, and/or caffeine.

- _____ is the best beverage for simple hydration.

- Drink when _____. The more _____ and _____ you eat, the less water you need.

- Fresh, homemade fruit and vegetable _____, liquid feed-me food, both hydrate and feed you.

Way to go! You've made it through breakfast, lunch, dinner, snacks, and beverages. Take it one choice, one day at a time. Just like all changes, eating better takes practice and patience. You not only can do it, you *are* doing it! Give yourself a big pat on the back.

"Eat the good guys _____ and the bad guys_____."

- Dr. Leslie Van Romer

Answer Key:

4. First, 10-veggie salad
   Second, steamed vegetables
   Third, potatoes, yams, rice, black
   Last, beef, chicken, fish, pasta
5. Am I full?, stop, vegetables
9. fruits, cut-up vegetables, raw, unsalted nuts and seeds
10. water, juices
11. juices
12. deplete

What You Now Know
- beef, chicken, pork, fish, pasta, bread
- 1. veggie
  2. vegetables
  3. vegetable, sweet, black
- 25%, fat
- deplete
- Water
- thirsty, fruits, vegetables
- juices

"Eat the good guys <u>first</u> and the bad guys <u>last</u>."

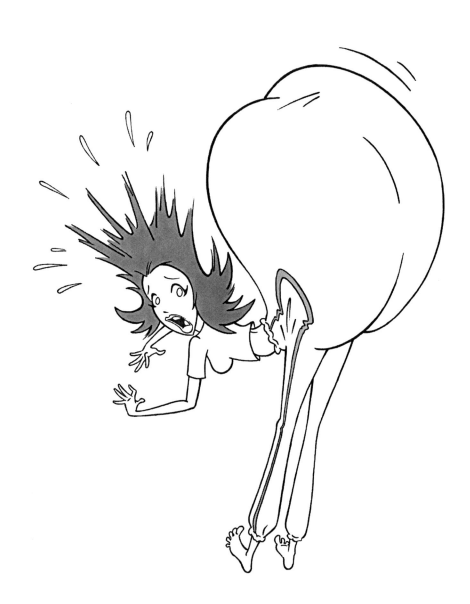

Chapter 10
21 "Big Buts" between You and Your Pants

1. "Big buts" that stop you from starting

    A. Yeah, but this way of eating is too _____.
    B. Yeah, but I get no _____ at home.
    C. Yeah, but I already eat a healthy enough diet, and I'm still _____.
    D. Yeah, but I don't like to be d_____ from other people.

2. "Big buts" that sabotage you along the way

    A. Yeah, but a little won't _____ me.
    B. Yeah, but I _____ sweets.
    C. Yeah, but I will get b_____ eating like this.
    D. Yeah, but there are _____ everywhere.
    E. Yeah, but I'm very social and love to eat in r_____ and with friends.
    F. Yeah, but I'm going on v_____ for a month.
    G. Yeah, but I get too much g_____ from fruit and veggies.
    H. Yeah, but losing _____ pounds a month is too slow.

3. Food-specific "big buts"

   A. Yeah, but if I don't eat meat, where do I get my _____?
   B. Yeah, but if I don't eat dairy, where do I get my _____?
   C. I don't like _____. (Fill in the blank with a food you don't like.)
   D. Yeah, but I love _____. (Fill in the blank with a deplete-me food.)
   E. Yeah, but what about vitamin _____?
   F. Yeah, but what about _____ in the blood?

4. Other people's "big buts"

   A. Yeah, but I don't have a chance. Everyone in my family is heavy – it's g_____.
   B. Yeah, but my spouse does the food _____ and makes the _____.
   C. Yeah, but my _____ won't eat like this.

5. Circle which "big buts" (listed in 1-4 above) are stopping you from getting into those pants. Are there any other "big buts" stopping you from filling up on feed-me foods 80% of the time? Write them below.

   _____
   _____
   _____
   _____

6. Are you ready to blast through those "big buts" to fill up on feed-me foods to lose weight and build your body-best? Yes ____ No ____

WHAT YOU NOW KNOW...

- "Big buts" are inevitable; their stopping you from getting into your pants is not.

> "You are the master of your own choices and either the beneficiary of or the slave to the consequences."
>
> - Dr. Leslie Van Romer

Answer Key:

1. A. radical
   B. support
   C. overweight
   D. different
2. A. kill
   B. crave
   C. bored
   D. temptations
   E. restaurants
   F. vacation
   G. gas
   H. 2.5
3. A. protein
   B. calcium
   E. B12
   F. anemia
4. A. genetic
   B. shopping, cooking
   C. spouse

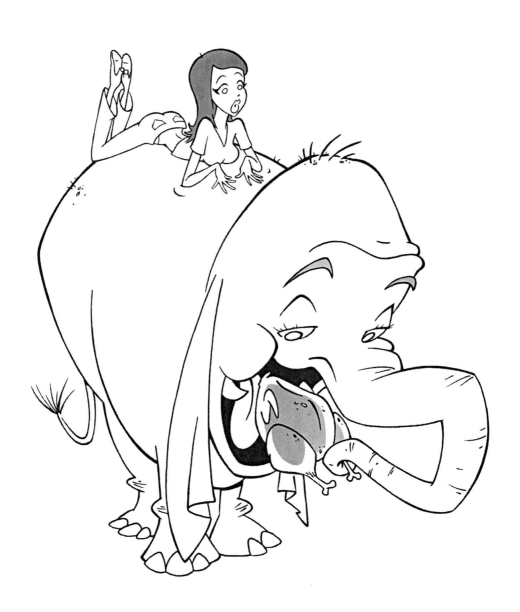

Chapter 11
Proteins, Plants, and Pants

"BUT WHERE DO I GET MY PROTEIN?"

1. Proteins can be compared to the _____ in a car.

2. Carbohydrates can be compared to the _____ that makes the engine run.

3. How much protein do you need?

    A. We grow the most from _____ to _____ year old.
    B. _____ _____ is the ideal food for babies.
    C. There is _____ % protein in breast milk.
    D. The World Health Organization says we need only _____ % protein for health.
    E. Oranges have _____% protein, tomato 16%, romaine lettuce 36% protein (yes! that much!), spinach 36%, broccoli 33%, cauliflower 26%, corn 11% (who doesn't like corn), potato 8%, carrot 9%, almonds 13%, pumpkin seeds 17%, brown rice 8%, oats 17%, kidney beans 27%.

4. The best sources of protein are whole _____ foods.

5. Animal protein comes packaged in animal foods, loaded with artery-clogging, disease-causing saturated fat and _____.

6. All _____ products contain cholesterol. In a 3.5 oz. serving, beef contains 85 milligrams of cholesterol, chicken 85 mg, pork 90 mg, trout 73 mg.

7. Plant foods contain _____ cholesterol. If your total blood cholesterol is 150 or below, you are virtually heart-attack proof.

8. Whole plant foods are naturally _____ in fat. Potatoes are 1% fat, broccoli 9% carrots 4%, romaine lettuce 10%, oranges 2%, apples 4%, brown rice 8%.

9. Animal protein alone, not counting the fat and cholesterol, is one of the most _____ substances that we eat. It contributes to heart disease, cancers (breast, colon, prostate), kidney diseases, and osteoporosis.

10. Elephants, giraffes, horses, and cows get their protein for great, big strong muscles from _____, not hamburgers, chicken, eggs, fish, or protein drinks.

11. "But where do I get my protein?" I get all the protein I need from _____.

WHAT YOU NOW KNOW...

- Proteins are critical for the structure, repair, maintenance, _____, and reproduction of cells and tissues.

- Protein is not the body's preferred _____ source, carbohydrates are.

- Plants, even just fruits and vegetables, provide plenty of _____ for the human body to thrive (oranges are 8% protein).

- Animal protein is associated with f___, ch_____, h_____, and c_____.

- Animal protein may be one of the most toxic, disease-_____ substances that we eat.

- When in doubt, look to _____ for answers. Where do elephants get their protein for great, big muscles? If they can eat _____ for protein, so can you.

> "Eating meat is a choice with consequences, not a necessity."
>
> - Dr. Leslie Van Romer

Answer Key:

1. engine
2. fuel
3. A. birth, one
   B. Breast milk
   C. 4.5%
   D. 4.5%
   E. 8%
4. plant
5. cholesterol
6. animal
7. 0
8. low
9. toxic
10. plants
11. plants

What You Now Know
- growth
- energy
- protein
- fat, cholesterol, hormones, chemicals
- causing
- nature, plants

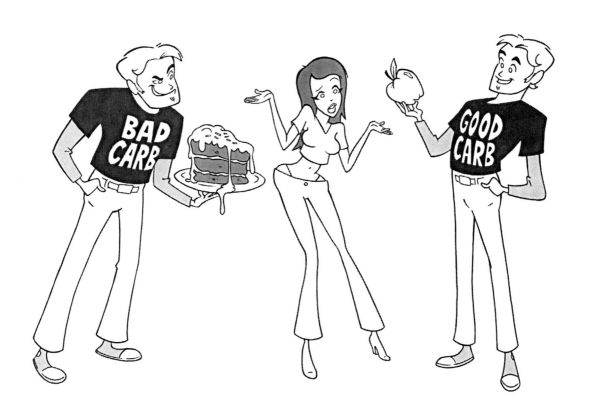

Chapter 12
The 20-Carb Solution into Your Pants

"BUT DON'T CARBS MAKE ME FAT?"

1. What are carbohydrates?
    A. Carbohydrates are the body's preferred _____ for energy.
    B. Whole _____ foods are the richest sources of carbohydrates.
    C. Meat and fish contain exactly ____% carbs, providing ____% energy.

2. Good carbs vs. bad carbs
    A. Good carbs, sourced by unrefined plant foods, boost health and energy, prevent _____, crush _____, satisfy _____ drive, and promote _____ loss.
    B. Bad carbs, found in refined white _____ and _____, are _____ in calories and are stripped of _____ and _____ for colon sweeping.
    C. Bad carbs trigger overeating, cravings, excess weight, _____addiction, aging, diseases, and a whole lot more.
    D. Both simple and complex carbohydrates can be either _____ carbs or _____ carbs.
    E. Fruits are made of simple carbohydrates that are _____ carbs.
    F. Refined, white flour, a complex carbohydrate, is a _____ carb.

3. How do you spot the bad-guy carbs?

   A. Read all _____ before eating any product.

   B. Refined sugars (bad carbs): sugar, brown sugar, corn syrup, rice syrup, dextrose, glucose, sucrose, lactose, maltose, fructose, dextrin, barley malt, "no sugar added," turbinado, evaporated cane juice, fruit juice concentrate, honey, and maple syrup.

   C. Breads are highly _____ foods. 99% of all breads have _____ flour. Breads are high in hidden s_____, refined flours, chemicals, oil, and sugar. They are not whole grains, but highly processed grains.

   D. Some of the _____ carbs are brown-colored _____ breads, rolls, pasta, muffins, bagels, tortilla shells, cereals, baked goods, cookies, cakes, pies, doughnuts, pastries, crackers, candy, chocolate, ice cream, frozen yogurt, jams, sugary drinks, soft drinks, canned foods, packaged foods, soups, spreads, salad dressings, ketchup, mayonnaise, pickles, spaghetti sauces, even baby foods - and that's certainly not all, folks.

WHAT YOU NOW KNOW...

- Your energy today is sourced by the good _____ from fruits and vegetables you ate _____.

- Good carbs are sourced by feed-me, whole _____ foods: fresh _____, fresh _____, whole _____, and _____.

- _____ carbs, empty of nutrition and high in calories, are sourced by refined and processed plant foods, as in _____ sugar and _____ flour.

- Read your _____!

GETTING INTO YOUR PANTS

"Proteins build your engine; carbohydrates provide
the fuel to make your engine run."

- Dr. Leslie Van Romer

Answer Key:

1. A. fuel
   B. plant
   C. 0%, 0%
2. A. disease, cravings, hunger, weight
   B. sugar, flour, high, nutrients, fiber
   C. food
   D. good, bad
   E. good
   F. bad
3. A. labels
   B. processed, white, salt
   C. bad, white
   D. label

What You Now Know
- carbohydrates, yesterday
- plant, fruits, vegetables, grains, beans
- Bad, white, white
- labels

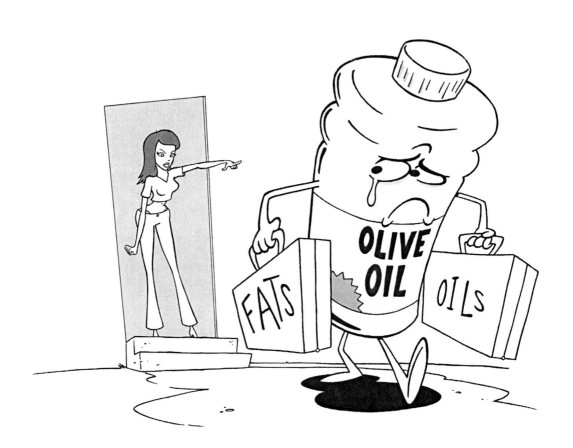

Chapter 13
Stop the Fats to Drop Your Pants (Size)

"BUT ISN'T OLIVE OIL A GOOD FAT?"

1. With the exception of two fats, all necessary fats are _____ by your body from the carbohydrates that you eat.

2. You need to eat very little fat and the two fats you do need to eat can come from a variety of _____ foods.

3. Olive oil is a good fat. True or False?

4. Added oils, including olive oil, offer you one thing only: extra fat to add to your fat. True or False?

5. The fat you eat is the fat you wear. True or False?

6. The worst kind of fat is too much fat. True or False?

7. Trans fats are altered fats or synthetic saturated fats found in hydrogenated fats, semi-solid oils. True or False?

8. Hydrogenated fats and trans fats cause heart disease, cancer, and diseases. True or False?

9. Local hang-outs for _____ fats and hydrogenated fats:

    Breads, fried foods, stick and tub margarines, butter substitutes, mayonnaise, shortening, spreads, dips, chips, crackers, cereals, salad dressings, peanut butter, chocolate, candy, pizza, processed foods, packaged foods, frozen dinners, packaged snack foods, energy/protein bars, vegetarian processed foods like soy burgers, pre-made diet meals, baked goods, like cookies, cakes, pies, desserts, microwaved popcorn, etc. . . .

10. Remember . . . fat goes from your lips to your _____ so get a grip.

WHAT YOU NOW KNOW...

- Fat is a major _____ needed for health.

- The worst kind of fat is too _____ fat.

- Your body _____ almost all the fats you need from the carbohydrates that you eat. (The two exceptions can be sourced by plants.)

- How much saturated fat and refined oils (including olive oil) should you eat? _____

- How much trans fat and hydrogenated fat should you eat? _____

- Whole _____ foods provide all the essential _____ you need.

"Extra cals are not your pals, gals."

- Dr. Leslie Van Romer

Answer Key:

1. made
2. plant
3. False
4. True
5. True
6. True
7. True
8. True
9. trans
10. hips

What You Now Know
- nutrient
- much
- makes
- none
- none
- plant, nutrients

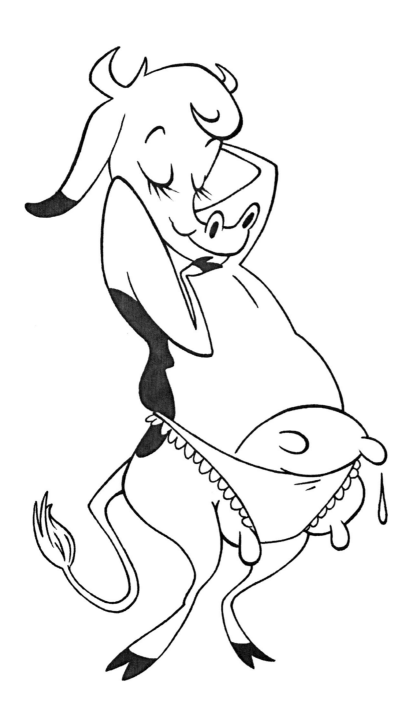

Chapter 14
Dairy's Dirty Underpants

"IF I DON'T DRINK MILK, WHERE DO I GET MY CALCIUM?"

1. Airing Dairy's Dirty Underpants

   A. Dairy products, like all animal products, contain saturated _____ and _____.

   B. Lactose, or milk s_____, causes indigestion, constipation, diarrhea, gas.

   C. Milk p_____, or casein, causes "little" problems: headaches, colds, sinus infections, earaches, allergies, bedwetting, pneumonia, depression, bronchitis, hyperactivity, asthma, eczema, mood swings, dripping nose, stuffiness, PMS, muscle pain.

   D. Milk p_____ is linked to huge problems: type 1 diabetes, lupus, arthritis.

   E. Some c_____ found in milk are bacteria, AIDS virus, leukemia virus, and pollutants from the environment.

   F. All meat, even organically raised meat, is overloaded with _____ that add to the human hormone level, which is related to hormonally-fed cancers: breast, prostate, pancreas, colon, and lung.

   G. Cows are given _____ to fight off udder infections caused by overuse and are artificially induced by artificial hormones to produce more _____.

   H. The government allows over 180 million ____ cells in one 8-oz glass of milk.

2. The Dairy-Cancer-Disease Connection: dairy is linked to killer cancers, strokes, types 1 and 2 _____, hypertension, Parkinson's, Crohn's, ulcerative colitis, irritable _____ syndrome, multiple sclerosis, lupus, atherosclerosis, rheumatoid _____, sinusitis, eczema, sniffing, and more . . . .

3. Revealing Calcium's Secret Stash

    A. The most direct, ideal sources of calcium are _____ foods.
    B. Cows get their calcium from _____, not from milk, cheese, or yogurt.
    C. Plants change _____ forms of calcium from the soil into _____ calcium for people and animals.

4. Osteoporosis: The Bone-Chilling Truth

    A. The U.S., England, New Zealand, Sweden, and Finland consume the most _____ products and have the highest rate of hip _____ from osteoporosis.
    B. Osteoporosis is caused by a negative _____ balance, more calcium leached out of bones than consumed.
    C. Osteoporosis is not a calcium-_____ disease. Americans eat plenty of calcium. They consume too many foods and non-foods that leach the calcium out of their bones.
    D. The biggest calcium robber of all is _____ protein.
    E. Other foods that leach calcium from the _____ are sugar, salt, soft drinks, alcohol, caffeine, smoking, and lack of _____-_____ exercise.
    F. Harvard study with 78,000 nurses showed that those who drank more milk suffered more fractures from _____.

WHAT YOU NOW KNOW...

- Drinking milk and eating dairy products are _____, not necessities.

- Fresh, whole _____ and _____ provide all the calcium we need.

- We are conditioned to eat and love _____. We're hooked on it.

GETTING INTO YOUR PANTS

- _____ products cause "little" problems: headaches, earaches, stomachaches, sniffing, sinusitis, congestion, colds, bronchitis, eczema, PMS, mood swings.

- _____ products are linked to big problems: cancer, heart disease, stroke, diabetes, hypertension, Parkinson's, Crohn's, ulcerative colitis, irritable bowel syndrome, multiple sclerosis, lupus, atherosclerosis, and rheumatoid arthritis.

- In this country, osteoporosis is not caused by the lack of _____. It is caused by what you eat that _____ the calcium out of your bones.

- Look to _____ for commonsense answers. Where do cows get their calcium to grow big bones and produce milk? _____, certainly not milk.

> "You are no more weak, lazy, or undisciplined than the rest of us mere mortals — you're simply a product of your conditioning."
>
> - Dr. Leslie Van Romer

Answer Key:

1. A. fat, cholesterol
   B. sugar
   C. protein
   D. protein
   E. contaminants
   F. hormones
   G. antibiotics, milk
   H. pus
2. diabetes, bowel, arthritis

3. A. plant
   B. plants
   C. inedible, usable
4. A. dairy, hip fractures
   B. calcium
   C. deficiency
   D. animal
   E. bones, weight-bearing
   F. osteoporosis

What You Now Know
- choices
- fruits, vegetables
- cheese
- Dairy
- Dairy
- calcium, leaches
- nature, plants

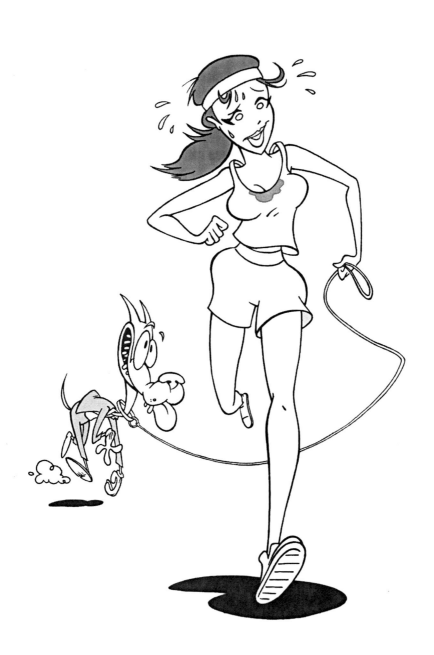

Chapter 15
Panting in Your Pants

"YEAH, BUT I HATE TO EXERCISE."

1. "Honestly, I am not exercising every day because _____
   _____."

2. From now on, I will follow the "D_____ S_____ Principle."

3. My self-created regular exercise routine:

   A. I like to _____ better than any other exercise.
   B. I will _____ this many days a week _____.
   C. I will _____ on alternate days.
   D. I will exercise _____ minutes per session.
   E. I will exercise at _____ o'clock every day or _____ days a week.
   F. I will go _____ to exercise.
   G. I will exercise with _____ to make it more fun.
   H. I will buy sneakers with excellent support, _____ control, and _____ bar.
   I. When I get off track, I will _____ to get back on track.
   J. I commit to _____ (kind of exercise), _____ days a week, for _____ minutes at a time, as well as _____ (kind of exercise) days a week, for _____ minutes at a time.

4. My great "big buts" blocking me from panting in my pants.

   Circle all that apply:
   A. But I don't have time
   B. But exercise is so inconvenient
   C. But I'm too tired
   D. But my husband won't walk with me
   E. But I have no place to exercise
   F. But I don't want to overdo
   G. But I exercise enough at work or home
   H. But it's too cold or hot or dark or…_____
   I. But it's been over 21 days, and I'm still fighting with it
   J. But I'm too lazy

WHAT YOU NOW KNOW…

- To add years to your life and life to your years, you've got to _____ your body.

- Just "D___ S_____" every day.

- Your biggest but that keeps you from firming up that jiggle when you wiggle is: _____.

- I am ready to blast through that "big but." I will not let it stop me from looking hot in those pants.

"Exercise doesn't take time, it gives you time when it counts — at the end of your life."

- Dr. Leslie Van Romer

Answer Key:

2. Do Something

What You Now Know
- move
- Do Something

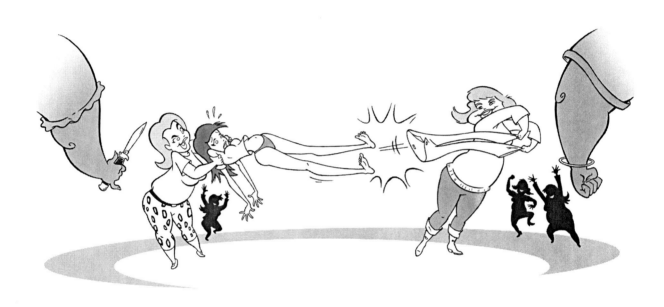

Chapter 16
7 Sneaky Sisters Stealing Your Pants

1. Name the 7 sneaky sisters:

   A. Wendy _____

   B. Frieda _____

   C. Patty _____

   D. Betty _____

   E. Annie _____

   F. Dena _____

   G. Greta _____

2. Which of the 7 sisters resemble you, and why? (Think hard about this!)

   _____
   _____
   _____
   _____
   _____
   _____
   _____
   _____
   _____

WHAT YOU NOW KNOW

- The biggest block between you and those pants: _____!

- Make the _____, hunker down, and f_____ t_____ with that do it or die determination – no matter which sisters nag you. With patience and persistence, you will get into those pants – a size _____ in a year.

> "Your outer world is the exact reflection of your inner world."
>
> - Dr. Leslie Van Romer

Answer Key:
1. A. Whiner
   B. Fear
   C. Perfect
   D. Bored
   E. Antsy
   F. Denial
   G. Greedy

What You Now Know
- you
- commitment, follow-through

Chapter 17 – Part I
The First Step into Your Pants

"HOW DO I GET STARTED?"

1. Your New-You Plan of Action.

    Okay – enough words. You've worked hard at learning 10+10 for Life® and a new way of thinking about food, weight loss, and building your body-dream-come-true. I hope you are amazed and proud of yourself for your vision, your commitment, and your determination to take action and follow through. I'm impressed, and so should you be. (Once more, what are the best weight-loss, feed-me foods? Fresh _____ and _____.)

    Now it's time to put your hard-earned knowledge into practice. Let's create a doable action plan to get you into those pants, shall we?

    Find a calendar to use for your plan-of-action. For your convenience, order your weight-loss *Pants Pocket Calendar* for $7.95 (in the U.S. and Canada), including postage and handling. E-mail info@drleslievanromer.com, and put "calendar" in subject line.

    A. Formulate your yearlong weight-loss goal and write it down on a calendar.

        Date: _____

        One-year weight-loss goal: _____ pounds. (I recommend no more than 30 pounds in a year – it's doable.)

Monthly weight-loss goal: _____ pounds. (I recommend 2.5 pounds a month – again, it's doable.)

One-year pants-size goal: _____. (I recommend about two sizes down.)

B. Write down your weight-loss goals on a separate piece of paper and put them in a visible place, like on the refrigerator or bathroom mirror or both. It will go something like this:

I will lose _____ pounds by _____ (date and year), exactly one year from today. That is exactly _____ pounds a month.

I will get into a size _____ pants by _____ (date and year).

C. Now record your weight and pants size on your starting month in the calendar. Record these two numbers at the beginning and end of each month for the next twelve months.

D. I suggest that you also write down at least five other yearlong goals that will improve with eating correctly (with wiggle room), exercising consistently, and losing weight. In the beginning of your *Pants Pocket Calendar,* there is a designated spot to record your goals.

Suggested goals:

1. Lower blood pressure
2. Lower cholesterol
3. Lower blood glucose and A1C
4. Get rid of aches and pains
5. Safely reduce or eliminate specific medications
6. Have the energy to work hard or play with your grandchildren
7. Renew enthusiasm for life
8. Engage in a certain favorite hobby or activity

9. Feel attractive
10. Enjoy sex again
11. Have fun shopping for clothes
12. Like the way your clothes fit
13. Feel good about yourself

What are your yearlong goals other than weight loss? Choose goals that are personal and relevant to you.

1. _____
2. _____
3. _____
4. _____
5. _____

E. Choose five specific action steps and write them down on the first month of your calendar. Your *Pants Pocket Calendar* provides a special place in the beginning and each month to write these action steps. If five is too many, then choose as many as you feel are reasonable for you. If five seems too few, *don't* add more. Stick to the five. It's very easy to take on too much, get totally overwhelmed, and then give up. No worries – you can add more action steps in the coming months. Start with five.

Here is an example of five common action steps.
1. Eat only fruit throughout the morning.
2. Eat daily a large, fill-me-up 10+10 salad for lunch.
3. Eat dinner in order with best-for-you foods first: salad, steamed vegetables, potato/winter squash topped with avocado/tomato/guacamole or rice and/or bean dish. *Stop* eating when full. Eat meat/fish/pasta last, if you must.
4. Eat fruit, cut-up veggies, and raw, unsalted nuts and seeds for snacks.
5. Walk at least four days a week for thirty minutes.

What are your five action steps for the first month? Choose action steps that are personal and relevant to you.

1. _____
2. _____
3. _____
4. _____
5. _____

F. Track your action steps on the calendar and congratulate yourself for all the things you do right. At the end of each day, write down the numbers that represent the specific action steps you completed on that day, right on the day in calendar.

For instance, if on Tuesday, April 1, 2008, you complete the first, second, fourth, and fifth action steps from your plan as I previously listed, simply write the number 1, 2, 4, and 5 on that day, April 1. This will help you:

1. Stay on track to reach your yearlong goals.
2. Keep a permanent record to refer back to when trying to figure out why you are or aren't losing as planned.
3. Feel good about YOU and everything you're doing for yourself.

G. Weigh yourself monthly and record your weight on the calendar.

H. Revisit the action steps every month to either delete, add, or change action steps. Keep these action steps very current and relevant. Remember to record the number of each action step you complete every day so you can give yourself those all-important, instant "atta-girls." This will take you no more than five seconds – do it!

I. At the end of the year, look at your original goals and completed action steps on every month of your calendar. Assess where you started, how far you've come, and where you want to go from here. Be proud of all of the action steps you completed and recorded with its number. Figure out your next year's goals and the next month's action steps.

2. Planning Your First Week of Meals. Take a look at the meals layed out for you in the book. Using those suggestions as a guideline, plan your week of meals which work for you. Then make your shopping list based on these meals.

Monday	Tuesday
· Breakfast _____, _____, _____, _____, _____, _____ (Examples: ¼ honeydew melon, 2 bananas, 2 oranges, 1 grapefruit, 2 apples, ½ cup of fresh raspberries) · Lunch _____ _____ _____ _____ Large 10+10 veggie salad with the following: several handfuls of chopped romaine lettuce, spinach, and arugula, ¼ sliced red onion, ½ avocado, a handful of shaved carrot slices (use a vegetable peeler to shave the carrots), ⅓ cucumber, 8-12 cherry tomatoes, 1 diced red bell pepper, a handful chopped raw broccoli. (Save a few large handfuls of undressed salad for dinner. Eat the rest.) Follow the salad, if and only if you still want it, with a slice of whole wheat toast topped with avocado or a chopped tomato. · Dinner_____ _____ _____ _____ 1. Eat the remaining 10+10 salad from lunch (add more lettuce and veggies if you want a bigger salad). 2. Steamed green beans and asparagus 3. Diced and steamed potato, topped with pureed avocado and/or fresh tomato salsa. Steam 1 extra potato for your lunch salad tomorrow.	· Breakfast _____, _____, _____, _____, _____, _____ (¼ pineapple, 2 apples, 4 plums, 1 nectarine, 2 peaches) ·Lunch_____ _____ _____ _____ Large 10+10 salad with red leaf lettuce, spinach, ¼ red onion, a handful of baby carrots, steamed, diced potatoes left over from the night before (potatoes really help fill you up, which is very important for weight loss and craving control), 1 green pepper, a handful raw cauliflower, 1 Roma tomato, ⅓ julienne zucchini, ⅓ chopped cucumber. If you're still hungry, eat asparagus left over from dinner or a handful of raw, unsalted, unsugared pecans. · Dinner _____ _____ _____ _____ 1. Cut-up cucumbers, red peppers, carrot sticks, cauliflower with avocado or hummus dip. 2. Black bean and brown rice burritos with tomatoes, shredded lettuce, jalapeños, onions, guacamole wrapped in whole wheat tortilla shell.

Wednesday	Thursday
· Breakfast _____, _____, _____, _____, _____, _____	· Breakfast _____, _____, _____, _____, _____, _____
(½ honeydew, 2 kiwis, 2 mangos, 1 nectarine, 1 pear, 2 oranges, grapes)	(Cooked whole oats with almond milk, blueberries, strawberries, raisins, apples, cinnamon, and a little raw honey – a reprieve from fruit only)
· Lunch _____	· Lunch _____
(100% sprouted-grain sandwich with avocado, tomato, red pepper, onions, cucumber, and hummus spread (a nice change-up from salad), and a handful of raw, unsalted almonds.)	(Eat the salad you made for dinner last night. If you are still hungry, enjoy a warm bowl of leftover lentil soup.)
·Dinner_____	· Dinner _____
1. Make enough salad for dinner tonight, and for your lunch tomorrow, with romaine and red leaf lettuce, arugula, carrots, cucumber, red pepper, zucchini, cauliflower, cherry tomatoes, green snap peas, sliced radishes, purple cabbage, and raw almonds. 2. Follow that with red lentil soup (see simple recipe). 3. If you are really hungry when you get to the soup, toast 1 slice of sprouted-grain bread to dip or steam a potato and pour the soup over the potato.	1. Again, make enough salad for dinner and lunch tomorrow, with romaine, red leaf, arugula, 1 avocado, cherry tomatoes, cucumber, zucchini, broccoli, shaved fennel from the bulb area, carrots, and raw, unsalted sunflower seeds. 2. Steamed broccoli and fennel (you can steam the bulb and the stems after slicing). 3. Black beans "stir-fried" in water with tomatoes, onion, chili powder, and cumin, topped with a little guacamole. Save some beans for next day's salad – beans are very filling.

Friday	**Saturday**
· Breakfast _____, _____, _____, _____, _____, _____	· Breakfast _____, _____, _____, _____, _____, _____
(2 bananas, 2 oranges, 2 apples, bunch of grapes, 1 mango, ¼ of your pineapple)	(¼ cantaloupe, 1 banana, 2 tangerines, 2 pears, grapes, the rest of your blueberries, strawberries, and raspberries or any other fruit you have left over)
· Lunch _____	· Lunch _____
(Eat the salad left over from last night, along with some of your leftover bean/vegetable mixture.)	(Make one large 10+10 salad to split between dinner and lunch with remaining lettuce, cucumber, carrots, Roma tomatoes, cherry tomatoes, broccoli, cauliflower, green and red peppers, and any other veggies lying around that look good to you. 2. If still hungry, make an open-faced, sprouted-grain sandwich with one slice of bread stacked with avocado, sprouts, lettuce, tomatoes, red peppers, and onions, spread with hummus.)
·Dinner_____	· Dinner _____
1. Make a salad with leftover lettuce and veggies and eat it while you cook, if you want to. 2. Steamed brown rice covered with a stir fry (in water or veggie broth) of broccoli, mushrooms, carrots, snap peas, zucchini, red onion, fresh ginger, and a bit of tamari sauce (like soy sauce). Top the veggies with finely chopped raw almonds and raw bean sprouts.	1. 10+10 salad leftover from lunch. 2. Spaghetti squash (excellent pasta substitute) topped with fresh tomato marinara sauce (see simple recipes in *Getting into Your Pants*).

Sunday

· Brunch with family: _____
_____
_____
_____

(Wiggle time! Sleep in and then eat whatever you want. You've earned it!)

· Afternoon snacks
_____
_____
_____

(raw, unsalted nuts and seeds, fruits, any leftover fruit.)

·Dinner_____
_____
_____
_____

1. 10+10 salad made of any leftover veggies. 2. Grilled portobello mushroom and yam topped with avocado puree and fresh tomatoes.

Notes

SHOPPING LIST

Fruits

_____   _____
_____   _____
_____   _____
_____   _____
_____   _____
_____   _____
_____

Vegetables

_____   _____
_____   _____
_____   _____
_____   _____
_____   _____
_____   _____
_____   _____

Fresh Herbs/Spices   **Grains/Beans**

_____   _____
_____   _____
_____   _____
_____   _____
_____   _____

Breads   **Other**

_____   _____
_____   _____
_____   _____
                               _____
                               _____

"It's not about being right; it's about doing what's right for you."

- Dr. Leslie Van Romer

Chapter 17 – Part II
Building Your Dream House

1. Did you have any ah-ha moments when you read *Getting into Your Pants*?
   Yes _____ No _____

2. If yes, what were they?
   A. _____
   B. _____
   C. _____
   D. _____
   E. _____

3. List five major things you learned about food and/or weight-loss that are important to you and your success.
   A. _____
   B. _____
   C. _____
   D. _____
   E. _____

4. Which foods are your weight warriors and health heroes?

   _____ and _____

5. List the three rules in 10+10 For Life®.
   A. _____
   B. _____
   C. _____

6. What do you like about 10+10 for Life®?
   A. _____
   B. _____
   C. _____
   D. _____
   E. _____

7. What do you dislike about 10+10 for Life®?
   A. _____
   B. _____
   C. _____
   D. _____
   E. _____

8. Will any of these dislikes interfere with your weight-loss and body-best success?
   Yes_____ No_____

9. List 5 groups of feed-me foods.
   A. fruits.
   B. _____
   C. _____
   D. _____
   E. _____

10. List 5 deplete-me foods that you like but choose not to eat anymore.
    A. _____
    B. _____
    C. _____
    D. _____
    E. _____

11. List 5 deplete-me foods that you like and continue to eat.
    A. _____
    B. _____
    C. _____
    D. _____
    E. _____

12. What insights did you learn about yourself and/or your relationship with food from reading *Getting into Your Pants*?
    A. _____
    B. _____
    C. _____
    D. _____
    E. _____

13. List eating and/or exercise habits you have decided to change. Example: eating fruit instead of buttered popcorn in the evening or instead of eating chocolate every day.
    A. _____
    B. _____
    C. _____
    D. _____
    E. _____

14. What are your biggest buts between you and getting into those pants?
    A. _____
    B. _____
    C. _____
    D. _____
    E. _____

15. Which big buts are you ready to let go?
    A. _____
    B. _____
    C. _____
    D. _____
    E. _____

16. What are you still confused about when it comes to you, food, weight loss, and/or building your body-best?
    A. _____
    B. _____
    C. _____

17. When people ask you one of the four most commonly asked questions, you can choose to sidestep the question or suggest that they read about that topic in the appropriate chapter in *Getting into Your Pants*. Or learn the simple, commonsense answers so you can respond with absolute confidence, stopping them dead in their tracks. This takes practice. See Addendum 5 for the answers to:

    1. If you don't eat meat, where do you get your protein?
    2. If you don't eat dairy, where do you get your calcium?
    3. But don't carbs make you fat?
    4. But isn't olive oil a good fat?

18. Describe in detail your vision of yourself exactly one year from today. How do you want to look and feel? What will you be doing? Describe your role in your relationships, work, hobbies, etc.

    _____
    _____
    _____
    _____

19. Describe in detail your vision of yourself exactly five years from today.
   _____
   _____
   _____
   _____

20. Do you believe that you will transform your one-year and five-year visions into reality? Yes _____ No _____

    If yes, hugs and kudos to you and congratulations.

    If no, hugs and kudos to you, too. But why not? The body and life you want is waiting. What's stopping you? _____
    _____
    _____

21. What will your exact words be in response to the first person who asks you, "How did you lose all that weight?"
    _____
    _____

    Don't justify. Don't judge. Don't preach. And learn to duck.

    It's not about being _____ – it's about doing what's _____ for you.

WHAT YOU NOW KNOW...

- How to create a doable, yearlong, weight-loss plan-of-_____. Congratulations!

- How to choose and track monthly _____ steps to _____ your one-year goals: "I will lose _____ pounds and get into a size _____ pants."

- How to simplify 10+10 food _____ and organize your _____.

- How to plan for one week of _____ + _____ meals.

- How to shed _____, inside and out, and do what's right for you to build your _____ house – your body and your life, for life.

Congratulations to you, my friend. You have completed *Getting into Your Pants* with its companion *Pants PlayBook*! You've played hard. Now go all the way. Above all else, you deserve to feel good about you. See you this same time next year – prancing in those cuter-than-heck pants.

> "You are beyond great — you are extraordinary!"
>
> - with respect and admiration from Dr. Leslie to the unique and beautiful you

Answer Key:

Chapter 17 – Part I
1. fruits, vegetables

Chapter 17 – Part II
4. fruits, vegetables
5. A. Add
   B. Stop
   C. Wiggle
9. B. vegetables
   C. sprouts
   D. raw, unsalted nuts and seeds
   E. homemade fruit and vegetable juices
21. I'm simply eating better by filling up on more fruits and vegetables.
    It's not about being <u>right</u> – it's about doing what's <u>right</u> for you.

Addendum I
7 Steps to Stay in Those Pants

1. You gotta **really** want it – to get into those pants and stay there. Make a commitment to yourself. Are you ready? Yes _____ No _____

2. Make a conscious choice to follow a plan and to get back on track after getting off track. (And you will get off track!)

    Are you ready to promise yourself to incorporate 10+10 for Life® into your life, allowing yourself wiggle room? Yes _____ No _____

3. Create, record, and revisit realistic yearlong weight-loss and body-best goals.

    Have you written down your goals and are you willing to take the time and make the effort to work toward these goals, knowing you can change them at any time? Yes _____ No _____

4. Create, record, and revisit 5 doable action steps every month.

    Have you written down your first month's action steps? Yes _____ No_____

    If yes, are you willing to write down your updated action steps every month so you can get into your pants? Yes_____ No _____

    If no, go do it! Get serious about getting into your pants.

5. Track your progress and be amazed at everything you do right.

    Are you willing to write down the number of the action steps you complete at the end of the day, each day? Yes _____ No _____

6. Read, read, read, and read some more. Build a rock-solid foundation of facts.

   Are you willing to continue to expand your level of awareness and build your foundation of facts? Yes_____ No _____

7. Seek a support person.

   Accountability is absolutely critical to your success. Find one person that you can trust and depend on to support you and your effort to get into those pants and stay there.

   _____ is my support person and gentle, loving whip to hold me accountable (usually not a spouse).

Addendum II
10 Top 10+10 Tips

1. Ask "Which foods prevent cancer?" Fresh fruits and vegetables.

2. When you are making food choices, ask yourself, "Does this food feed me or deplete me?" See feed-me, deplete-me chart. If it feeds you, pat yourself on the back. If it depletes you, decide whether or not to eat that food.

3. Think addition, not subtraction. Think which foods do I "get to" add to my day instead of which foods do I "have to" give up.

4. Follow three 10+10 rules:
   - **Add:** Fill up *first* on fresh, whole fruits and vegetables. Shoot for 10 whole fruits and 10 different vegetables a day.
   - **Stop:** Stop eating when your brain says satisfied and full.
   - **Wiggle! (if you must):** Follow the 80/20 rule. Eat 80% feed-me foods. Give yourself 20% wiggle room to eat what you want (no more!).

5. Eat when you're hungry. Stop eating when you're full.

6. Snack on fruit, vegetables, raw, unsalted nuts and seeds. Always keep feed-me snacks with you.

7. Don't eat fruit with other foods.

8. Leave at least two hours between the time you last eat and the time you go to bed.

9. Clean out cupboards, throw away deplete-me foods, reorganize kitchen, and shop for feed-me foods. Ban the "bad guys" from your house and keep them out.

10. To lose weight, shift thinking, choices, habits, and lifestyle. Be patient and kind to yourself. Transitioning to your ideal weight and body-dream-come-true takes time.

"Fruits and vegetables: your weight warriors and health heroes."
– Dr. Leslie Van Romer

Addendum III
A 10+10 for Life® Food Day at-a-Glance

Breakfast

- Fresh, whole fruit only until 1 hour before lunch – enough to fill you up
- Second option: whole oats

Lunch

- Large, 10-veggie, green-leafy salad – enough to fill you up
  Eat first 80% of time.
- Salad dressing: organic vinegar of choice, ½ lemon, and diced avocado or an oil-free, dairy-free dressing
- Second options: vegetable sandwich with sprouted-grain bread or no-dairy, no-meat soup

Dinner

- Eat in order with best-for-you, feed-me foods first
- First, large, green-leafy salad – 10 raw veggies
- Second, vegetables steamed, baked, stir-fried (in water)
- Third, more filling vegetables, like potatoes, yams, or winter squash
  Topping: pureed avocado, tomato, onion, lemon, herbs; fresh tomatoes or salsa

  or

Whole grain, like brown rice or homemade legume dishes, like kidney or black beans

Stop and ask yourself, "Am I full?" If yes, stop eating. If no, choose to eat more vegetables or a more traditional dinner food.

- Last, eat traditional dinner foods or not at all (meat, fish, pasta)

Snacks

- Fresh fruit, veggies, raw, unsalted nuts, and raw, unsalted seeds

"With every bite, ask yourself, 'Does this food feed me or deplete me?'"
– Dr. Leslie Van Romer

Addendum IV
The 4 Most Common Questions and the Commonsense Answers

1. **"If you don't eat meat, where do you get your protein?"**

   Answer #1: What is protein for? Simply stated, protein is for growth. When do we grow the most? From birth to one year old. When do we need the most protein? From birth to one year old. What is the best food for growing babies? Breast milk. How much protein is in breast milk? 4.5% protein. That's all!

   Not coincidentally, the World Health Organization recommends 4.5% protein in our diets for human health. Oranges have 8% protein, broccoli 45% protein, romaine lettuce 36% protein, brown rice 8 % protein, kidney beans 26% protein. Plant foods give us plenty of protein, without the fat and cholesterol that come with animal protein. Two more protein points: 1. Plant protein is not inferior to animal protein. 2. Plant proteins don't have to be mixed and matched to make a "complete" protein.

   Answer #2: Look to nature for commonsense answers. Where do cows, horses, giraffes, and large elephants get their protein to grow and maintain big, strong muscles? They don't eat cows, pigs, lambs, chickens, fish, eggs, protein bars, or protein drinks. They eat unrefined plant foods, and not a huge variety at that. If they can get plenty of protein from plants, so can we.

2. **"If you don't drink milk or eat cheese, where do you get your calcium?"**

   Answer #1: Plant foods. Where do cows, horses, giraffes, and elephants get their calcium for strong bones and teeth? Plants. They certainly don't drink milk (once weaned) and another mammal's milk at that. Cow's milk is made for baby cows, not for baby people much less grown-up people. Period. The only milk made for baby people is mama's milk.

Answer #2: Unrefined plant foods contain all the nutrients you need, including calcium. Nature is so smart. Where does calcium come from? The soil. Calcium is dissolved in water in the soil and absorbed by plants. Plants transform inedible, unusable calcium from the soil into usable calcium needed by all mammals. Eating plants is the most direct way of getting calcium, and without the fat, cholesterol, animal protein, milk sugar, hormones, antibiotics, other toxins, and pus (yes, pus!), which come in dairy products.

3. **"But don't carbs make you fat?"**

Answer: All carbohydrates are not created equally. There are good carbs and bad carbs. Good carbs are sourced by whole, unrefined plant foods, as in fruits, vegetables, grains, and legumes, the best-for-you foods. The good carbs you ate yesterday give you the fuel for your body and your energy today. (No, protein doesn't give us energy.)

Bad carbs are sourced by refined plant foods, such as white sugar and white flour products – breads, cookies, pastries, doughnuts, cake, candy, desserts, soft drinks, store-bought drinks, and many processed, packaged foods. Too many calories from bad carbs are changed into fat, adding fat to your fat.

4. **"But isn't olive oil a good fat?"**

Answer #1: Your body makes all the fats it needs, with only two exceptions, which are sourced by a variety of plant foods. Therefore, it serves no purpose whatsoever to add more fat to the ready-made fat, especially a highly concentrated, refined fat that comes without any nutrition. All added oils, even olive oil, offer you one thing only: calories, and those calories come with a fat price tag – more fat added to your hips, tummy, thighs, and arms. That makes olive oil a bad fat.

Answer #2: Look to nature for simple answers. Where do elephants get their necessary fats? Olive, canola, or flax seed oil? Of course not. Plant foods provide all of our essential nutrients, including fats. Grapefruits contain 2% fat, oranges 4% fat, oatmeal 15% fat, broccoli 9% fat, apples 4% fat, romaine lettuce 10% fat, and cabbage 6% fat.

> "You've got nothing to lose — except weight — and everything to gain — like life."
>
> – Dr. Leslie Van Romer

Addendum V
Charts

WEIGHT CHART FOR WOMEN

According to this chart, at my present weight of _____ pounds, I am approximately _____ pounds overweight. At this time next year, I will weigh _____ pounds and get into a size _____ pants.

Weight in pounds, based on ages 25-59 with the lowest mortality rate
(wearing indoor clothing weighing 3 pounds and shoes with 1" heels)

Height	Small Frame	Medium Frame	Large Frame
4'10"	102-111	109-121	118-131
4'11"	103-113	111-123	120-134
5'0"	104-115	113-126	122-137
5'1"	106-118	115-129	125-140
5'2"	108-121	118-132	128-143
5'3"	111-124	121-135	131-147
5'4"	114-127	124-138	134-151
5'5"	117-130	127-141	137-155
5'6"	120-133	130-144	140-159
5'7"	123-136	133-147	143-163
5'8"	126-139	136-150	146-167
5'9"	129-142	139-153	149-170
5'10"	132-145	142-156	152-173
5'11"	135-148	145-159	155-176
6'0"	138-151	148-162	158-179

"Losing weight is a shedding process – from the inside out."

– Dr. Leslie Van Romer

GETTING INTO YOUR PANTS

WEIGHT CHART FOR MEN

According to this chart, at my present weight of _____ pounds, I am approximately _____ pounds overweight. At this time next year, I will weigh _____ pounds and get into a size _____ pants.

Weight in pounds, based on ages 25-59 with the lowest mortality rate
(wearing indoor clothing weighing 5 pounds and shoes with 1" heels)

Height	Small Frame	Medium Frame	Large Frame
5'2"	128-134	131-141	138-150
5'3"	130-136	133-143	140-153
5'4"	132-138	135-145	142-156
5'5"	134-140	137-148	144-160
5'6"	136-142	139-151	146-164
5'7"	138-145	142-154	149-168
5'8"	140-148	145-157	152-172
5'9"	142-151	148-160	155-176
5'10"	144-154	151-163	158-180
5'11"	146-157	154-166	161-184
6'0"	149-160	157-170	164-188
6'1"	152-164	160-174	168-192
6'2"	155-168	164-178	172-197
6'3"	158-172	167-182	176-202
6'4"	162-176	171-187	181-207

CALCULATING YOUR FRAME SIZE

Following is the method the Metropolitan Life Insurance Company uses to calculate frame size:

1. Extend your arm in front of your body bending your elbow at a ninety degree angle to your body so that your forearm is parallel to your body.
2. Keep your fingers straight and turn the inside of your wrist towards your body.
3. Place your thumb and index finger on the two prominent bones on either side of your elbow. Then measure the distance between the bones with a tape measure or calipers.
4. Compare to the chart below. The chart lists elbow measurements for a medium frame. If your elbow measurement for that particular height is less than the number of inches listed, you are a small frame. If your elbow measurement for that particular height is more than the number of inches listed, you are a large frame.

Elbow Measurements for Medium Frame			
Men	Elbow Measurement	Women	Elbow Measurement
5'2" - 5'3"	2-1/2" to 2-7/8"	4'10"-4'11"	2-1/4" to 2-1/2"
5'4" - 5'7"	2-5/8" to 2-7/8"	5'0" - 5'3"	2-1/4" to 2-1/2"
5'8" - 5'11"	2-3/4" to 3"	5'4" - 5'7"	2-3/8" to 2-5/8"
6'0" - 6'3"	2-3/4" to 3-1/8"	5/8" - 5'11"	2-3/8" to 2-5/8"
6'4"	2-7/8" to 3-1/4"	6'0"	2-1/2" to 2-3/4"

"Body first, everything else second."

– Dr. Leslie Van Romer

BODY MASS INDEX

According to the BMI chart on the following page, my BMI is _____.

      I am (circle one)…

      Underweight

      Normal weight

      Overweight

      Obese

      Extremely obese

With my BMI of _____ and waist size of _____, my risk for getting a disease is (see Risk for Diseases chart, page 100):

      No increased risk

      Increased

      High

      Very high

      Extremely high

By this time next year, I will drop my BMI to 24 or less, normal BMI, and my waist size to _____, so I can get into a size _____ pants.

DETERMINING YOUR BODY MASS INDEX (BMI) AND RISK FOR DISEASE

To use the BMI table below, find your height in the left-hand column. Move across the row to your weight. The number at the top of the column is your BMI. BMI can overestimate body fat in people who are very muscular and underestimate body fat in people who have lost muscle mass, such as the elderly.

BMI (kg/m²)	19	20	21	22	23	24	25	26	27	28	29	30	35	40
Height (in.)	Weight (lb.)													
58	91	96	100	105	110	115	119	124	129	134	138	143	167	191
59	94	99	104	109	114	119	124	128	133	138	143	148	173	198
60	97	102	107	112	118	123	128	133	138	143	148	153	179	204
61	100	106	111	116	122	127	132	137	143	148	153	158	185	211
62	104	109	115	120	126	131	136	142	147	153	158	164	191	218
63	107	113	118	124	130	135	141	146	152	158	163	169	197	225
64	110	116	122	128	134	140	145	151	157	163	169	174	204	232
65	114	120	126	132	138	144	150	156	162	168	174	180	210	240
66	118	124	130	136	142	148	155	161	167	173	179	186	216	247
67	121	127	134	140	146	153	159	166	172	178	185	191	223	255
68	125	131	138	144	151	158	164	171	177	184	190	197	230	262
69	128	135	142	149	155	162	169	176	182	189	196	203	236	270
70	132	139	146	153	160	167	174	181	188	195	202	207	243	278
71	136	143	150	157	165	172	179	186	193	200	208	215	250	286
72	140	147	154	162	169	177	184	191	199	206	213	221	258	294
73	144	151	159	166	174	182	189	197	204	212	219	227	265	302
74	148	155	163	171	179	186	194	202	210	218	225	233	272	311
75	152	160	168	176	184	192	200	208	216	224	232	240	279	319
76	156	164	172	180	189	197	205	213	221	230	238	246	287	328

RISK OF DISEASES ACCORDING TO BMI AND WAIST SIZE

Risk of Associated Disease According to BMI and Waist Size			
BMI		Waist less than or equal to 40 in. (men) or 35 in. (women)	Waist greater than 40 in. (men) or 35 in. (women)
18.5 or less	Underweight	--	N/A
18.5 - 24.9	Normal	--	N/A
25.0 - 29.9	Overweight	Increased	High
30.0 - 34.9	Obese	High	Very High
35.0 - 39.9	Obese	Very High	Very High
40 or greater	Extremely Obese	Extremely High	Extremely High

"You deserve to feel good about you."

- Dr. Leslie Van Romer

TRACK YOUR NUMBERS

Write down your numbers from your last physical and today's number on your own scale. Get these numbers from your health practitioner if you don't know them. With your doctor's help and support, track your numbers every three months for the next full year. Your numbers speak volumes.

Date_____

Weight_____   Height_____   Age_____
Body Mass Index (BMI)_____   Blood Pressure_____   Total Cholesterol_____
Blood Glucose_____   A1C_____   Triglycerides_____

Date_____

Weight_____   Height_____   Age_____
Body Mass Index (BMI)_____   Blood Pressure_____   Total Cholesterol_____
Blood Glucose_____   A1C_____   Triglycerides_____

Date_____

Weight_____   Height_____   Age_____
Body Mass Index (BMI)_____   Blood Pressure_____   Total Cholesterol_____
Blood Glucose_____   A1C_____   Triglycerides_____

Date_____

Weight_____   Height_____   Age_____
Body Mass Index (BMI)_____   Blood Pressure_____   Total Cholesterol_____
Blood Glucose_____   A1C_____   Triglycerides_____

"Be the hero of your body-dream-come-true."

- Dr. Leslie Van Romer

Printed in the United States
143576LV00004B/1/P